SMURFS™

THE LOST VILLAGE

Popcorn
ELT
Readers

SMURF VILLAGE

TEAM SMURF

Clumsy

Smurfette

Smurfy selfie!

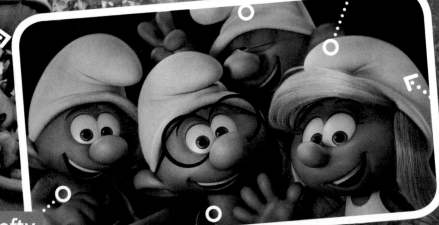

Hefty

Brainy

Smurfs wear white hats.

THE ENCHANTED FOREST

Papa Smurf

The Enchanted Forest is a magic place.

You mustn't go into the Enchanted Forest. It's dangerous!

Gargamel wants to catch the Smurfs. He wants their magic. A long time ago, Gargamel made Smurfette.

Monty

'Now catch the Smurfs for me!' he said to Smurfette. But Papa Smurf saw the good in Smurfette and the Smurfs were soon her friends.

Gargamel the wizard

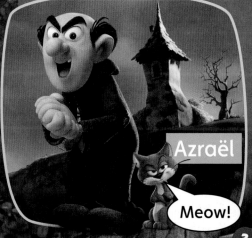

Azraël

Meow!

Before you read ...
What do you think? Who or what lives in the Enchanted Forest?

© Peyo

New Words

What do these new words mean? Ask your teacher or use your dictionary.

© Peyo

arrow

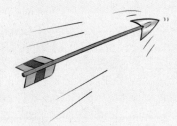

This is an **arrow**.

catch

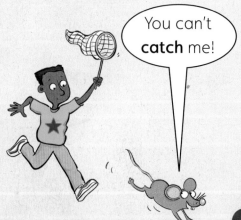

You can't **catch** me!

cauldron

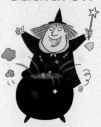

She has a big black **cauldron**.

dragonfly

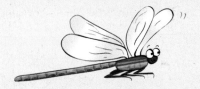

This **dragonfly** is blue.

freeze

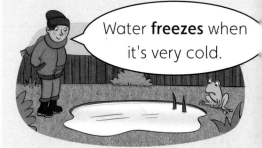

Water **freezes** when it's very cold.

magic

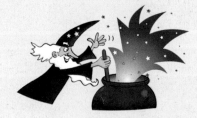

The wizard is making **magic**.

raft

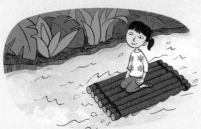

She is sitting on a **raft**.

river

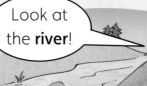

Look at the **river**!

real

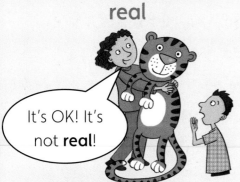

It's OK! It's not **real**!

save

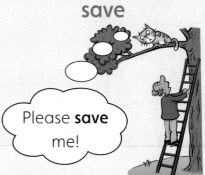

Please **save** me!

'do the right thing'

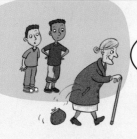

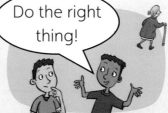

Do the right thing!

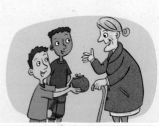

What does the title *The Lost Village* mean? Ask your teacher.

Verbs

Present	Past
fall	fell
fly	flew
take	took

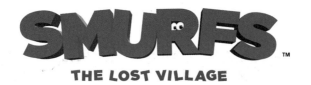

SMURFS™
THE LOST VILLAGE

CHAPTER ONE
The small brown hat

It was dark in Gargamel's house. There was one small light. It came from the cauldron.

Gargamel took something out of the cauldron. 'Look at this!' he said to his friends, Azraël and Monty. 'It's my first freeze-ball!'

'Meow!' said Azraël.

'I'm going to catch the Smurfs with these freeze-balls!' said Gargamel.

Azraël looked for Smurfs.

'Meow!' said Azraël. He could see some Smurfs.

'Quick!' Gargamel shouted to Monty. 'Catch them!'

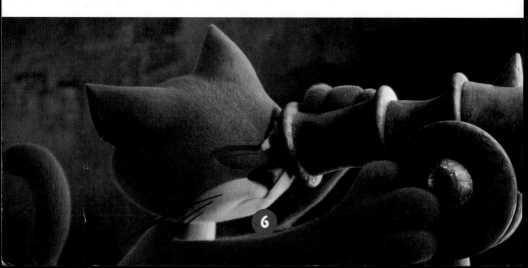

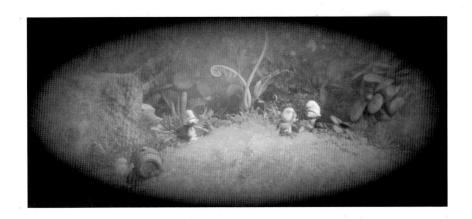

Smurfette and her friends liked to play near the Enchanted Forest.

'This is great!' said Clumsy. 'We are Team Smurf!'

Smurfette laughed. It was good to be with her friends.

Suddenly, something moved. Smurfette looked and some Smurf eyes looked back at her.

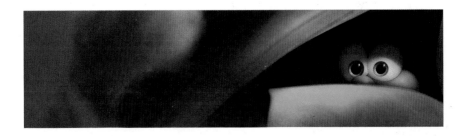

'Who are you?' asked Smurfette.

The Smurf ran away. It ran into the Enchanted Forest.

'Wait!' shouted Smurfette. 'Don't go!'

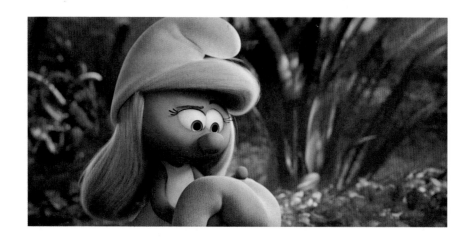

'Who was it?' asked Clumsy.

'I don't know,' said Smurfette. 'It ran away.'

Smurfette saw something near her feet. It was a small brown hat.

'CAW-CAW!'

Suddenly, Monty flew down. The friends were very frightened.

Monty took Smurfette and flew away.

'Stop!' shouted Hefty. 'Smurfette!'

But Smurfette was far away.

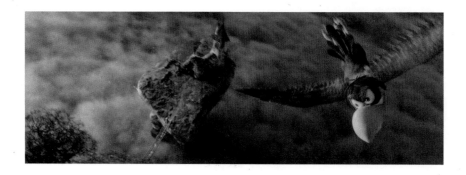

Monty flew back to Gargamel's house.

'Yes!' shouted Gargamel. 'A Smurf!'

Then he saw Smurfette.

'Oh no!' he said. 'Not you! You're not a real Smurf!'

Smurfette was quiet. She had the brown hat in her hand. Gargamel saw it.

'What's that?' he asked.

Gargamel put the hat into his cauldron.

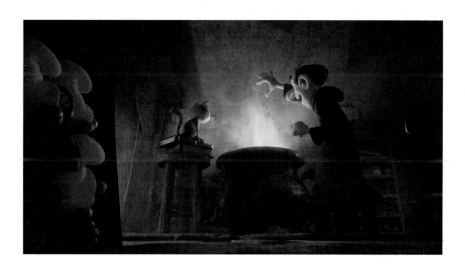

'Whose hat is this?' he asked.

The cauldron answered:

> Look in the forest - a magic place!
> But can you see a Smurfy face?
> Look in the forest to find their home!
> The Smurfs are there in Smurfy Grove!

'Aha!' Gargamel shouted. 'Let's go to Smurfy Grove!'

Smurfette's friends were behind Gargamel. He didn't see them. They saved Smurfette.

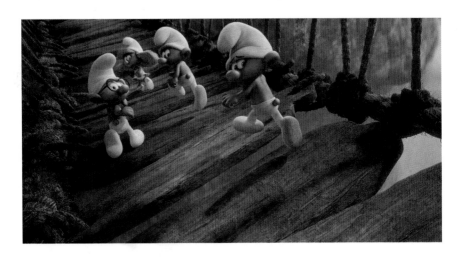

Team Smurf ran quickly back to Smurf Village.

'We have to stop Gargamel!' said Smurfette to Papa Smurf. 'We have to go to the Enchanted Forest and find Smurfy Grove.'

Papa Smurf didn't like that idea. 'You mustn't go into the Enchanted Forest,' he said. 'It's dangerous!'

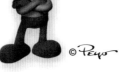

CHAPTER TWO
Team Smurf!

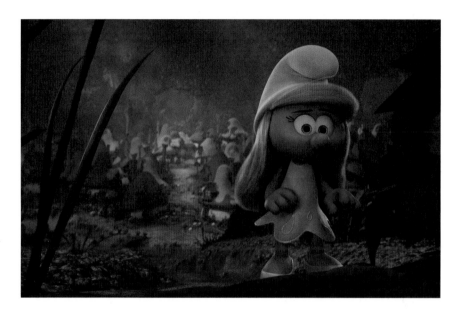

That night Smurfette did not sleep. 'Gargamel knows about Smurfy Grove,' she thought. 'I have to find it. I have to help the Smurfs there.'

Smurfette walked quietly out of the village. It was very dark near the Enchanted Forest. Suddenly, there was a noise behind her.

'Who is it?' asked Smurfette.

'We're coming too!' said Hefty.

It was Team Smurf!

The four friends were frightened but they walked slowly into the Enchanted Forest.

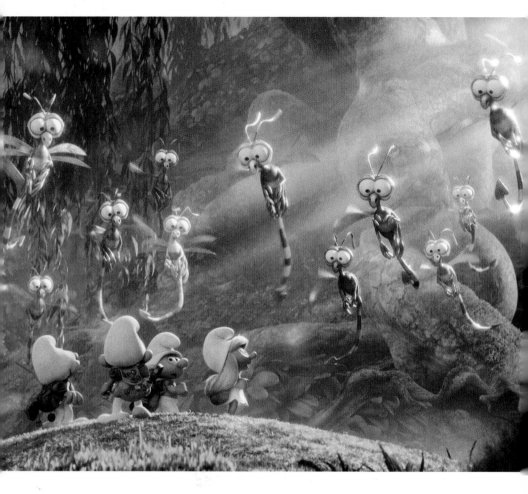

'Wow!' said Smurfette. 'It's beautiful!'

'Look at these dragonflies!' said Brainy.

'THAT dragonfly is very big!' said Clumsy.

But it wasn't a dragonfly. It was Monty. And Gargamel was behind him.

'Run!' shouted Hefty. The Smurfs ran and ran.

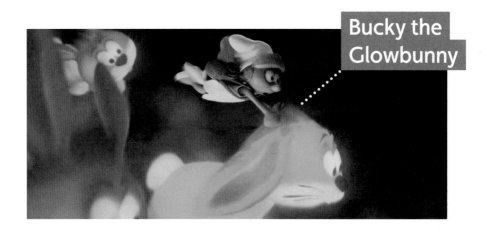

Bucky the Glowbunny

Suddenly Smurfette saw Bucky the Glowbunny.

'Quick!' shouted Smurfette. 'Jump on!

Bucky ran into the forest.

'Yes!' shouted Smurfette. 'Go Team Smurf!'

It was a big forest. Bucky ran for a long time.

'Let's stop to eat,' said Hefty.

The Smurfs were tired. But they were happy and they were friends.

'Smurfy selfie!' said Brainy.

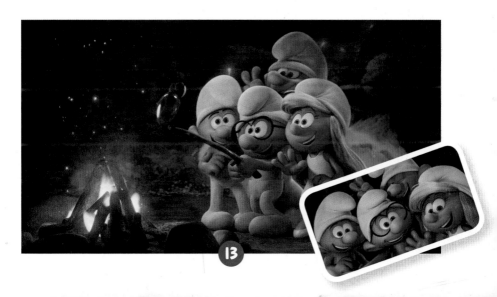

CHAPTER THREE
Smurfs do the right thing!

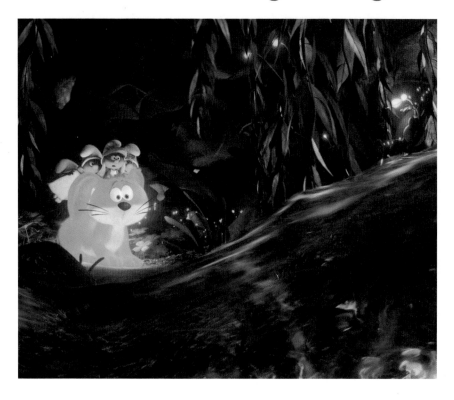

'Come on!' said Smurfette. 'We can't stay here.'

Bucky and the Smurfs walked all night. Suddenly, Bucky stopped. It was a river.

'Not a problem!' said Brainy. 'But I need some help from Team Smurf.'

The Smurfs helped Brainy.

'Wow!' said Smurfette. 'A raft! You are clever!'

'Let's go!' shouted Hefty.

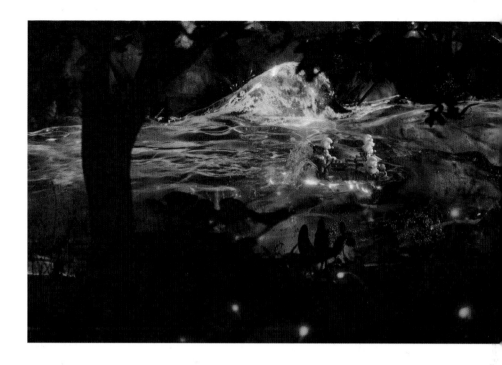

The river was fast.

'We're very near to Smurfy Grove now,' said Smurfette.

'HELP!'

'Who's that?' said Clumsy.

It was Gargamel. He was in the river with Azraël and Monty.

'We have to help him!' said Hefty.

'No!' said Brainy. 'It's Gargamel!'

'HELP!' shouted Gargamel again.

'I don't want to help him,' said Smurfette. 'But we're Smurfs and we do the right thing.'

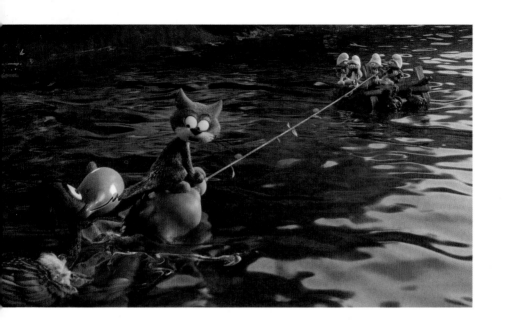

The Smurfs saved Gargamel.

'Thank you, Smurfs!' said Gargamel.

The Smurfs looked at Gargamel. Gargamel looked at the Smurfs.

'Great raft!' said Gargamel.

Suddenly, he jumped up and all the Smurfs fell into the water.

'I'm Gargamel and I'm bad!' he shouted.

CHAPTER FOUR
Smurfy Grove

When Smurfette opened her eyes, she was next to the river.

'I'm OK,' she thought. Her friends were OK too, but they were not happy.

'I want to go home,' said Brainy.

WHIZZ!

'What was that?' said Hefty.

WHIZZ! WHIZZ!

'Arrows!' shouted Brainy. 'Help!'

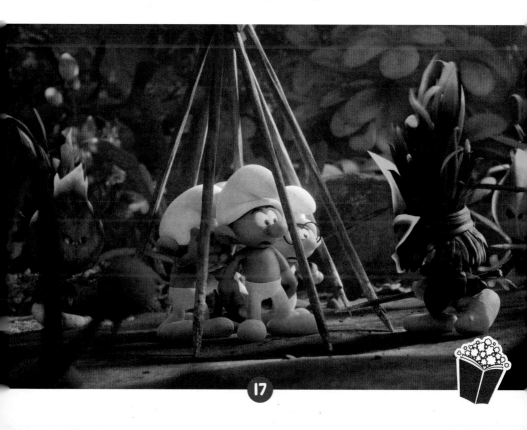

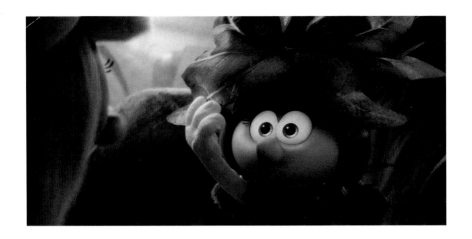

'It's OK!' said Smurfette. 'Look! Smurfs!'

'I'm Smurflily and this is Smurfstorm,' said one of the Smurfs. 'Who are you?'

'I'm Smurfette,' said Smurfette. 'You're girl Smurfs! There are only boy Smurfs in Smurf Village.'

Smurfstorm looked at Smurfette's friends.

'Boys?' she asked. 'What are boys?'

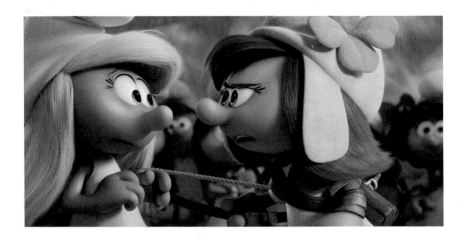

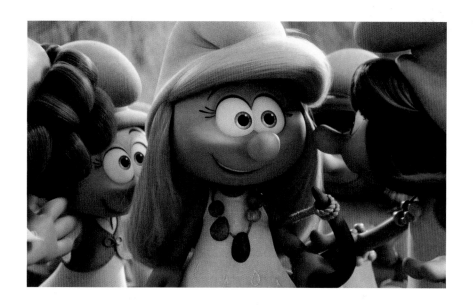

The girl Smurfs took Smurfette and her friends back to Smurfy Grove. Smurfstorm flew on a dragonfly.

'I love it here!' said Smurfette.

But Smurfstorm was not happy. 'Why are you here?' she asked.

'We want to help you,' said Smurfette. 'Gargamel is coming to Smurfy Grove.'

'Garga-who?' asked Smurfstorm.

'He's a wizard,' said Clumsy. 'He makes bad magic.'

'We need to find him,' said Smurfstorm. 'Come on!'

'Me?' said Clumsy. 'OK ...' He jumped on the dragonfly.

Smurfstorm and Clumsy flew over Smurfy Grove. They flew over the river.

'That's Gargamel!' shouted Clumsy. 'He made Smurfette.'

'He's very near Smurfy Grove,' said Smurfstorm. 'Quick!'

Smurfstorm and Clumsy flew back to the Smurfs.

'He's here!' shouted Smurfstorm. 'And Smurfette's not a real Smurf! Run!'

'No!' shouted Smurfette. 'I'm your friend!'

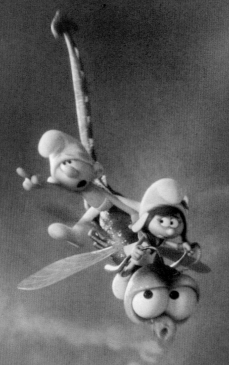

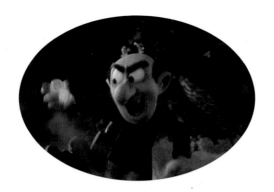

'FREEZE-BALL!' shouted Gargamel. 'FREEZE-BALL!'

Freeze-balls flew at the Smurfs. They could not move. Gargamel put the Smurfs in his bag.

'One Smurf for me!' he said. 'And one more Smurf for me!'

But he did not put Smurfette in the bag.

'Come on, Azraël,' he said. 'Let's go!'

'Gargamel found Smurfy Grove because of me,' Smurfette said sadly.

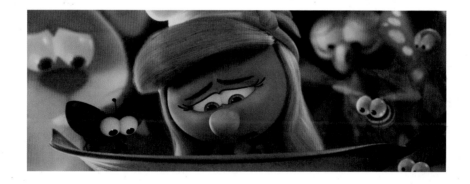

She looked at the selfie of Team Smurf.

'But Smurfs always do the right thing!' she said.

CHAPTER FIVE
All the magic!

At Gargamel's house, Gargamel took the magic from the Smurfs.

'Now I'm very strong!' shouted Gargamel. 'And I'm young again! I'm going to have all the magic!'

Smurfette walked in. 'Not ALL the magic!" she said.

'YOU again! Why are you here?' asked Gargamel.

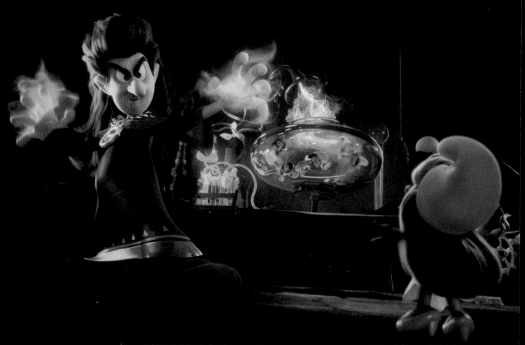

'You made me,' said Smurfette, 'and I took you to Smurfy Grove. But you don't have all the Smurfs and you don't have all the magic. I can take you to Smurf Village. Give me your magic. I want to be bad like you.'

'No, Smurfette!' shouted her friends.

'All the Smurfs?' said Gargamel.

'Yes!' said Smurfette.

'All the magic?' said Gargamel.

'Of course!' said Smurfette.

'You can have the magic,' he shouted. 'Be bad, Smurfette!'

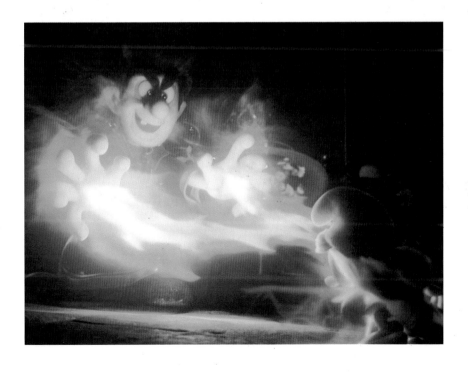

Smurfette took the magic from Gargamel.
But Smurfette was strong. She did not want to be
bad. Now there was a lot of magic in Gargamel's
house. The Smurf magic was stronger than
Gargamel.

'No!' shouted Gargamel. 'What are you doing,
Smurfette?'

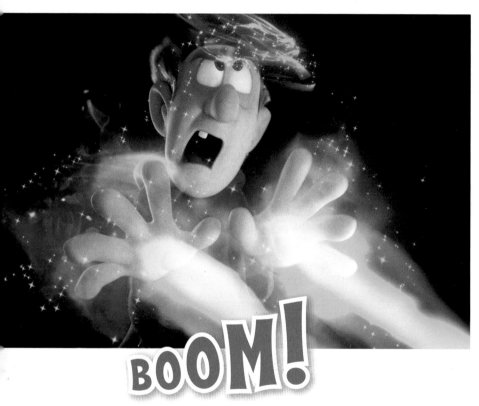

BOOM!

Gargamel flew out of his house. He flew far
away from the Enchanted Forest and far away
from Smurf Village.

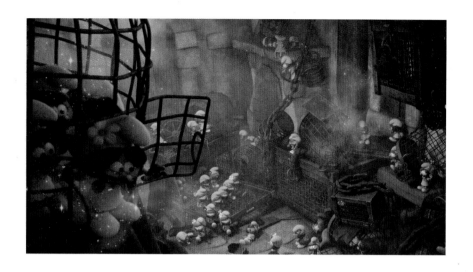

'You saved us!' laughed the Smurfs. 'Thank you, Smurfette!'

'You can come to Smurfy Grove every day!' said Smurfstorm.

'You are very strong!' said Hefty.

'You are a real Smurf!' said Clumsy.

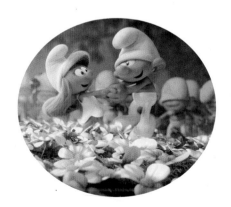

THE END

AMAZING DRAGONFLIES

The dragonflies in the Enchanted Forest are beautiful, but they are also dangerous. How much do you know about dragonflies in the real world?

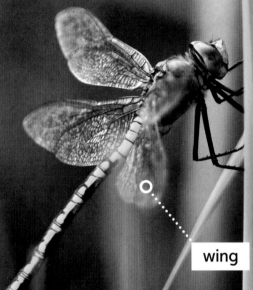

wing

Fast and strong

Dragonflies are very good at flying. They have four wings. They can fly backwards too. Dragonflies only fly on sunny days.

Look at those eyes!

Dragonflies' eyes are very big. They can see other flying insects - and catch them! Dragonflies eat a lot of mosquitoes.

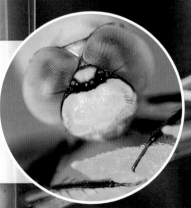

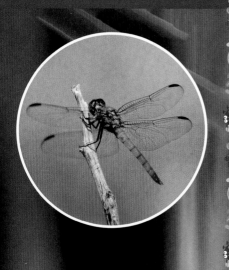

DID YOU KNOW?

Dragonflies were one of the first insects on Earth. The first dragonflies lived 350 million years ago. The first dragonflies were very big and had very long wings.

Underwater larvae

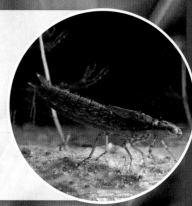

You can often see dragonflies near water. Their larvae, or babies, live underwater. The larvae can't fly but they can hunt! They are dangerous and they eat a lot of different insects. They live underwater for two years.

What do these words mean?
Find out.

amazing   backwards   insect
mosquito/mosquitoes   hunt

Where can you see dragonflies near your home?

After you read

1 Circle the correct word.

a) *Smurfy Grove* / *Smurf Village* is in the Enchanted Forest.

b) The *boy* / *girl* Smurfs live in Smurfy Grove.

c) The Enchanted Forest *is* / *is not* beautiful.

d) *Brainy* / *Gargamel* makes a raft.

e) The Smurfs *save* / *do not save* Gargamel from the river.

f) Gargamel catches the Smurfs with *arrows* / *freeze-balls*.

g) *Azraël and Monty* / *Smurfs* do the right thing.

2 Read these facts about Smurfette. Are they true (✓) or false (✗)? Write in the box.

a) Gargamel made her. ✓

b) Gargamel is her friend. ☐

c) She wears a small white hat. ☐

d) She took Gargamel to Smurf Village. ☐

e) She wants to be bad. ☐

f) She is a good friend. ☐

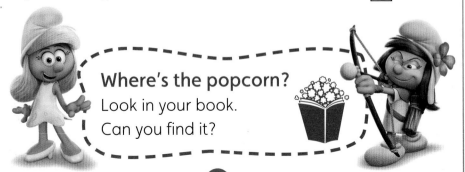

Where's the popcorn?
Look in your book.
Can you find it?

Puzzle time!

1 Answer the questions.

an arrow   a freeze-ball   a cauldron

a raft   a hat

Which of these ...

a) ... is very cold?   ....a freeze-ball..........

b) ... can fly?   ....

c) ... is very hot?   ....

d) ... can you wear?   ....

e) ... goes on water?   ....

2a How much can you remember? Answer the questions.

How many ...

a) ... dragonflies are there in the picture on page 12? `11`

b) ... animals does Gargamel have? ☐

c) ... Smurfs are in the Smurfy selfie? ☐

d) ... boy Smurfs are there in Team Smurf? ☐

e) ... girl Smurfs are there in Smurf Village? ☐

2b Now check your answers.

© Peyo

3a Who is this? Read about and draw the Smurf.
Write the name.

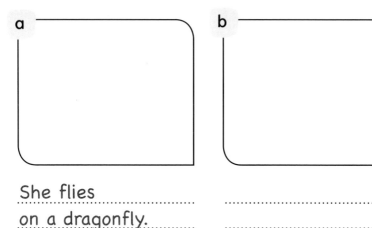

a _____

b _____

She flies
on a dragonfly.

It's .... !

....

....

It's .... !

3b Draw and describe a new Smurf.

4 Do you like these characters from the story?
Why? / Why not?

a) Brainy is my favourite. He's very clever!

b) ....

c) ....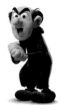

d) ....

Imagine ...

1 Work with four friends. Choose a character.
Read the dialogue.

Smurfette	We're very near to Smurfy Grove now.
Gargamel	HELP!
Clumsy	Who's that?
Hefty	We have to help him!
Brainy	No! It's Gargamel!
Gargamel	HELP!
Smurfette	I don't want to help him. But we're Smurfs and we do the right thing!
Gargamel	Thank you, Smurfs! Great raft! I'm Gargamel and I'm bad!

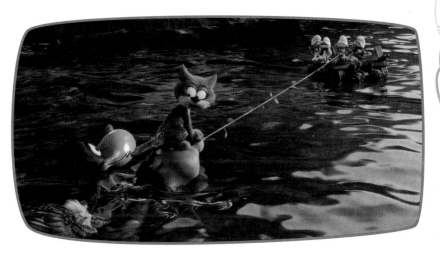

2 Act out the scene.

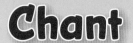

Chant

1 **T 9** Listen and read.

Look in the forest!

Look in the forest -
A magic place!
But can you see
A Smurfy face?

Look in the forest
To find their home!
The Smurfs are there
In Smurfy Grove!

Look in the forest -
Smurfette's there too!
But who can win?
Smurfette or you?

T 10 Say the chant.

© Peyo